Contents

Foreword

Ranald Boot

When you study the health issues that are prevalent in our society today and read the research that is published, there is only one conclusion you can arrive at:

We are causing most of our ill health ourselves!

We are literally buying food that poisons us. Then when we get sick we expect doctors to cure us with pills and potions from pharmaceutical companies. These just mask the symptoms of headache or arthritis or acid reflux, etc. and do nothing about the underlying causes. By taking the medicine we may feel better but we are not made well. The problems are still there and while we continue to eat the same foods they won't go away, our health will continue to decline.

Studies not only show how we can cure people from illnesses, they also tell us that the people showing an illness are the 'tip of the iceberg'! They may have had an overload of the source of the problem or a genetic predisposition to a problem but this doesn't mean the rest of us are ok. If we are all eating the same things we too will have some of the illness or damage caused by the very same foods. Our bodies are doing a marvellous job to keep us appearing 'normal' but over the years this fight puts severe strain on them. We are less resistant to infections and illness. We age faster, we have higher medical costs, our enjoyment of life is diminished and because it is happening to many others around us we think it is normal.

Our health system should be called a disease management system. If a visit to a doctor made us well, then the doctor would suffer financially because we would not return every month for more pills.

By any standards our health is declining, our brains are 10% smaller than they were 100 years ago. Spending on anti-depressants in the USA in 1985 was about $250 million, today it is over $14 billion! I could go on but there are some valid reasons for our declining health. The first is the dependence on a low fat high carbohydrate diet. The second is the cumulative effect of succeeding generations of poor nutrition following what doctors, dieticians and the Heart Foundation told us was good for us. Each following generation incurs more problems – more ADHD, more diabetes, more infertility, etc. and thirdly our food continues to be manipulated and contaminated by scientists to raise output and saleability at the expense of nutrition.

As individuals we can accept this situation and suffer the consequences, or we can learn what our bodies need and must have for optimum health. We have to accept total responsibility for our life and the choices we make. Our health is more than 70% determined by what we eat and drink. So if you get sick you, or someone else in the case of children, have made the wrong food decisions! Life is not a trial run, we can see what today's food and recommended diet is doing to us. The only way to prevent and overcome illness is with food choices. Either go with the flow and get sicker, or change and flourish.

In her book, Ann has brought together lots of valuable information along with recommendations that are easy to understand and follow. Doing so will enable us to experience the amazing benefits available from feeding our body the food it needs. So let's learn how to keep ourselves and our families well for as long as possible.

Introduction

Can many of today's illnesses really be caused by the food we eat, and if so, why are we not racing to do something to change it. What is it that's stopping us?

Too many young people today are suffering from obesity, diabetes, auto-immune disorders, celiac disease and associated problems. Can we blame this on our diet? So much of the food we are advised to eat as a 'Healthy Choice' doesn't look that way when you check the ingredients and find large quantities of sugar, salt, preservatives, flavour enhancers, thickeners, hydrogenated vegetable protein, colouring, sulphites, an array of numbers and more. Reading the back of the packet should put us off completely but no, the print is so small and the packaging so alluring, the ingredients addictive, so into the trolley they go.

For many years we have been encouraged to eat 'Low Fat/High Carb' processed food but this diet is not the way we humans were originally designed to eat. After reading further you too will find that the foods we thought were good for us are actually causing a whole lot of problems. These foods are production and media driven rather than health driven and marketed to look so good sitting on the supermarket shelf. It seems ridiculous to think they could possibly harm us.

Fact: Our body is designed to burn fat. This has always been its primary preferred fuel. So why is our modern life-style encouraging us to eat a Low Fat/High Carb diet?

Fact: Natural Fat is not bad for us, it contains many essential nutrients, satisfies our hunger, and eaten in moderation does not cause our body to gain weight.

Fact: Sugar is in all our processed food. It is not a dietary requirement and our bodies struggle to deal with it. It is poisoning us but we love it.

Fact: Today's so called 'Healthy Diet' is based on 'Grains', overloading our bodies with carbohydrates. When digested they turn into glucose triggering the release of insulin into our blood stream. Insulin stores the glucose as fat in our muscles, liver and around our internal organs and waist.

The change from burning fats for energy, as our ancestors did, to burning carbohydrates for energy as our modern diet dictates, is resulting in the decline of our health and the increase of obesity, diabetes, heart disease, auto-immune problems and coeliac disorders. If we really want to do something to reverse this trend, loose the spare tyre around our belly and restore our body to overall 'Good Health', the answer is simple. **Stop eating all grains**, and **drastically reduce** or preferably eliminate most other **carbohydrates**. "Crazy" you say, well read on.

My aim in writing this book is to make available to you the remarkable facts I have discovered. I hope they will spur you on, as they did me, to change your diet and reap the benefits. You will be amazed how your overall health improves and how effortlessly you regain your optimum weight. After reading "Primal Body, Primal Mind", by Nora Gedgaudas, my partner and I decided to change our diet back to one similar to our 'Hunter Gather' ancestors just for a month to see how we felt. That was over a year ago and the change in our health is remarkable. Nothing will make us go back to our old diet. Please read on because with a little determination there is no reason why a change in diet wouldn't work just as well for you. If you have health problems or just want to lose weight but can't, or think you are doing great at present but eating a Low Fat/High Carb diet, your health is a ticking time bomb. The earlier you change the healthier you will be.

There are many informative books out there on this subject and as I am sure after reading this you will want to learn more I have suggested some of them, along with interesting web sites, throughout this book.

*   *   *   *   *   *   *

Chapter 1

Our Diet – where it all started

We humans are genetically the same as our ancestors of around 40,000 years ago. We are still 'Hunter Gatherers' but nowadays for most of us our hunting is done in Malls and our gathering in Supermarkets. Most of our food is grown, processed and packaged for us. We have become the targets of product advertising, buying and eating food whether it is good for us or not.

History: It is estimated that humans have inhabited the earth for 2.5 million years. During this time the earth has gone through many ice ages with long periods of extreme cold in most regions and arid dry desert conditions in others. These ice ages were interspersed with relatively short warmer times; the most recent of these began about 20,000 years ago and provides us with the warm climate we enjoy today. [i]

Studies of fossilized human faeces from between 300,000 to 50,000 years show a lack of evidence of plant material suggesting that our ancestors existed for a considerable amount of our early evolution on only the meat and fat of the animals they found or caught.[ii] To survive on this diet and in extreme conditions their bodies burnt fat as its primary fuel.

Genetics: Around 10,000 years ago it is believed that eating grains and legumes became for many 'Hunter Gatherers' a way of surviving lean hunting. Their ability to use fire as a means of cooking made this sort of vegetation less toxic and therefore survivable but it wasn't as nutritious as animal meats. It was only 2,000 years ago that agriculture as we know it was established in Europe. Scientists believe it takes between 40,000 to

100,000 years for our body's genetic make up to adapt to such a significant change in diet. (Gedgaudas 2009-11)

So in human evolutionary terms preference for grains and legumes over meat is extremely recent. It is no wonder that our digestive system has problems coping with this type of diet, even with our food industry's ability to highly process them.

Fats and **Carbohydrates:** Fat is and has always been our body's preferred fuel. We were designed to eat animal meats, fish and other sea food, birds and eggs, nuts and berries, all with varying amounts of beneficial fats, vitamins and minerals easily accessed by our digestive system.

The 'Agricultural Revolution' brought large amounts of grains into our diet. Grains are high carbohydrate food; technically they are just chains of sugar molecules. Our bodies can manufacture sugar (glucose), as needed for our red blood cells or for any flight or fight situation, from a combination of protein and fat. We have no actual dietary requirement for carbohydrates in order to be healthy. When we fuel our bodies with carbohydrates instead of protein and fat, we are overloading our bodies with glucose. Do this on a constant daily basis and we create problems, our bodies just can't cope, we send ourselves down the road to obesity, diabetes and many other diseases.

What would happen if we could go back to eating a diet similar to our 'Hunter Gatherer' ancestors?

*　*　*　*　*　*　*

Chapter 2

Food Pyramids

Our modern day food pyramid is heavily weighted with grains. When I researched food pyramids that encouraged us to eat 'Healthily', most looked like this:

Fats, Oil, Sweets

Milk, Cheese, Yoghurt

Meat, Poultry, Fish, Beans, Eggs, Nuts

Vegetables, Fruits, Legumes

Bread Cereals Grains Pasta Rice

It does point out that "Sweets", and presumably sugary foods are not good for us but then it hasn't taken into account that the whole recommended bottom line of the pyramid turns into sugar (glucose - triglycerides) once digested.

If we take what our ancestors ate and put it into a food pyramid it would look like this:

Grains Legumes (in lean times)

Nuts, Fruits, Berries

Starchy Vegetables

Fibrous Vegetables

Game Meat Fish Birds Eggs Seafood

Our genetic made up is still very much the same as our 'Hunter Gatherer' ancestors for whom dietary fats, especially omega 3 fatty acid, played a very big part not only in their survival but in the rapid development of their brains. Fat is the body's most efficient burning fuel, it is essential for many bodily processes the most important being fuel for the brain.

Scientists have found that our brains have decreased in size by 10% over the past 100 years and believe the lack of essential fatty acid in our diet has been the biggest contributor to this.[iii]

So why are we being told, to be healthy, we should eat a 'Low Fat' diet with lots of grains and starchy vegetables when for most people it clearly isn't working?

* * * * * * *

Chapter 3

Healthy Whole Grains I don't think so!

Many plants, including the grains and legumes we eat today, contain toxic compounds designed by nature to prevent animals and insects from eating them.

Grains and legumes contain **'Phytic acid'** which deplete our bodies of minerals such as; calcium, iron, magnesium and zinc; **'Goitrogens'**, which are thyroid-inhibiting substances, causing an underactive thyroid, hypothyroidism; **'Exorphins'** which create cravings; and **'Gluten',** modern wheat having the highest level of gluten of all the grains.

Gluten is made up of two protein families, gliadin and glutenin. It is the gliadin proteins that trigger the immune response causing the damage in coeliac disease.[iv] Gluten makes flour doughy and elastic, great for bread making but not so for the human digestive tract. Gluten sensitivity is more widespread than we realise. Over time it causes the lining of our small intestine to become 'threadbare' and permeable. This is often called **'Leaky Gut'** and gives us all sorts of problems. Gluten is a major cause of many of our modern illnesses including heart disease and cancer.[v] You don't have to be diagnosed with coeliac disease before noticing gluten's impact on your health. Just stop eating grains to experience how much brighter and fitter you feel.

Grains are also very **starchy carbohydrates** and when broken down by our digestive system turn into sugars, namely 'glucose' causing our blood sugar levels to quickly rise and our pancreas to produce insulin. The worst grain is **wheat**, "two slices of 'Healthy Whole Grain Bread' will raise our blood sugar levels higher and quicker than a sugary drink, a candy bar or two tablespoons of sugar", says William Davis, MD, author of 'Wheat Belly'.[vi] Davis goes on to explain that today's wheat is very different to the grain our ancestors managed to gather. Our wheat has been hybridized and turned into a super carbohydrate with less protein and fibre and more gluten. When digested it triggers a set of inflammatory disorders, an addictive response and of course excess glucose levels.

What this means is our **'Healthy Whole Grain'** products such as bread, pasta, breakfast cereals, etc. are putting us all on the path to **Obesity**, **Diabetes**, **Coeliac disease** and **Coeliac like disorders**, via their gluten and carbohydrate content. If you eat grains, especially wheat, you will have these problems to some degree and could also suffer from the following.

- Migraine headaches, Chronic fatigue.
- Shortness of breath, Anaemia.
- Rheumatoid Arthritis, Osteoporosis.
- Irritable bowel syndrome, Ulcerative colitis.
- Rashes, Acne, Hives.
- Thyroid problems, Tiredness, Weight gain.
- ADHD, Autism, Learning Difficulties.
- Brain Fog, Dementia, Alzheimer's, Parkinsonism.
- Allergies, Dermatitis, Diary intolerance.
- Lung complaints, Cancer.
- Auto immune diseases, MS, Chron's disease.
- Neurological symptoms, Ataxia, Depression.
- Peripheral neuropathy, Gluten encephalopathy.
- Miscarriages or Infertility.
- Obesity, Visceral fat around internal organs.

Wheat products are as addictive as sugar or alcohol because they contain **'Exorphins'.** These cause the addictive response in our brain. They are opiate-like peptides that produce cravings. The more we eat the more we want.

Eliminating grain from our diet will lessen the yoyo effect of blood sugar rise and fall, suppress our appetite, and stop the accumulation of belly fat. It will also lower blood pressure if needed, reduce inflammation throughout our body and improve bowel health.

 Continuing to eat a high carb/low fat diet that includes lots of grains, will only lead to those illnesses mentioned above.

 "We can start to rectify this and become healthier simply by stopping eating Grains!"

*   *   *   *   *   *   *

Chapter 4

Carbohydrates - just another name for Sugar

Remember, to remain healthy we have NO dietary requirement for carbohydrates.   All grains, even 'Healthy Whole Grains', starchy vegetables, sweet fruits and all foods containing sugar of any sort, when eaten cause our blood glucose to rise. This forces our pancreas to produce insulin and release it into the bloodstream in order to quickly remove the glucose from our blood. Every time we take a mouthful of bread, eat a piece of cake or bite into pastries, snack bars, a bag of crisps, an ice-cream, drink a can of coke/juice or a glass of wine, this process will occur. Some of the glucose is used for energy as a way of getting rid of it but most is transferred into the cells of our muscles and liver or deposited as fat around our waist (visceral fat). Then the level of blood glucose drops and we feel hungry again. The constant high/ low glucose level is very damaging to our body as our pancreas is repeatedly producing insulin.

When our cells are continually exposed to high levels of insulin they become desensitized, and fail to accept the glucose out of our bloodstream. The pancreas then pumps out more insulin still attempting to lower our glucose. Continue to eat a 'High Carb/Low Fat' diet and our pancreas can't keep up, our blood sugar continues to rise and we become a **Type II diabetic.**

High sugar levels also start a process known as **'Glycation'**, (advanced glycated end products – AGE for short) where sugars react with the protein and fat within our blood stream forming AGEs. This debris causes hardening and clogging of our arteries, damages our tissues and collects in our kidneys, liver, skin, eyes (cataracts) and joints (arthritis). It mucks up our neurological pathways causing dementia, heart disease and strokes. **Our body can't get rid of AGEs and the damage done by glycation is mostly irreversible**. Prevention is the best solution. Giving up sugary carbohydrates is a great place to start.

Consuming carbohydrates at all or most meals will ensure that our body burns sugar for its energy requirements, surplus will be stored as fat and our existing stores of fat will not get used. We gain weight, tire quickly, often feel hungry or crave comfort foods, get easily stressed, experience brain fog, have high fasting triglycerides levels, our bones become brittle and eventually we become insulin resistant (diabetic). **When we put an end to chronic carbohydrate consumption our body uses dietary and body fat as its fuel** – great for weight loss, our blood glucose is stable and we can go many hours without feeling hungry, our insulin levels remain low causing little to no damage to our body.

How many carbohydrates do you think you consume in a day?

Breakfast: cereal (grains and sugar), 'Healthy Whole Grain' toast and jam, crumpets, bagels etc; Morning tea - a biscuit, scone, muffin or snack bar.

Lunch: sandwiches, filled bread rolls, flat bread, pies and sausage rolls, etc.

Coffee and tea: with sugar, soft drinks, energy drinks, fruit juices or a smoothy.

Dinner: pasta, potatoes, kumara, carrots, and/or any starchy root vegetable, also rice, couscous, corn tacos, noodles. Battered fish and anything deep fried.

Dessert: a smorgasbord of sugary delights.

That's just the basics, what about all those in-between snacks, sweets, peanuts and dried fruits, chocolate bars, muesli bars, crisps, even large amounts of fresh fruit – anything more than a handful of berries and there's another big sugar (glucose and fructose) load spiking your insulin and stressing your liver. If all, or some, of this sounds familiar to you and you can tick these boxes then you are definitely a carbohydrate burner, dependent on sugar, requiring frequent feeding and continuous insulin production.

Carbohydrates and Sugar are the most unnecessary and damaging of all foods we eat. They are the hardest to give up because they are so Addictive!

*   *   *   *   *   *   *

Chapter 5

Goodbye Grains and Sugar

Change from being a sugar burner to becoming a fat burner. Aim for a higher fat/low carb diet. Consuming a regular amount of dietary fat means you won't feel hungry and you will have more energy. The associated protein we consume will be used for our body's structural repair and maintenance. Our insulin production can go back to doing its intended job of coordinating our energy stores to match our life-span and reproduction.[vii]

Start by avoiding all wheat and wheat containing foods, and severely limit sugary food. Use the 'Hunter Gatherer's' food pyramid as well as the lists below as a guide. Work towards eating no grains at all simply because it is not just the gluten we are trying to avoid.

Foods to avoid - to keep blood sugar levels stable, avoid visceral fat and glycation:

All grains – wheat and wheat flour products, oats, quinoa, sorghum, buckwheat, millet, barley, corn, rice and foods made from starches, corn flour, potato flour, rice flour, arrowroot and tapioca.

Legumes – beans – all varieties, chickpeas, lentils, split peas, green peas, humus dips and spreads, peanuts, peanut butter (peanuts are not nuts).

Drinks – ideally avoid or seriously limit, fruit juices, energy drinks, sugary soft drinks, low calorie soft drinks, wine, beer, spirit mixes, milkshakes, yogurt drinks and artificial sweeteners.

Snack foods – all the so called healthy snack bars because they are full of grains and sugar. Biscuits, cakes, slices and cracker biscuits, rice biscuits etc. All processed foods with their associated man made fats, often called 'trans-fats'.

All sugary deserts – commercial ice-cream, most flavoured yogurts and large quantities of fresh fruit.

Vegetables oils – all commercial oils, all food cooked in commercial oil.

Beware Gluten free foods – as they will have used cornstarch, rice starch, potato starch, tapioca starch, arrowroot powder and other very refined carbohydrates in place of wheat flour.

Foods to eat - to maintain a healthy body:

Meat and Protein - grass fed beef, lamb, pork, venison, chicken, turkey, duck, fish, eggs, cheese (cultured or fermented), nuts, some seeds, with all their associated saturated fat.

Vegetables – all fibrous vegetables (mainly those grown above ground), leafy greens and salads greens, avocados, tomatoes and cucumbers, onions, leeks, courgettes, celery, pumpkin etc. Eat only very small amounts of starchy vegetables like - kumera, parsnip, carrots but not potatoes – as they originate from the 'nightshade' family.

Oils – coconut, cold press olive and nut oils, (cook with coconut oil as it doesn't degrade with heat).

Fruit – small amounts of berries are best as they have the lowest glucose levels. Most fruit today has been breed to be very sweet. Search for low GI fruits, like berries, kiwi fruit and gooseberries.

Desserts – a small amount of blueberries with a dollop of coconut cream sprinkled with chopped walnuts. Once your body is burning fat for fuel you will find you won't crave deserts.

Try going Grain and Sugar free for a week, then two or three maybe a month. You will be delighted with the results.

Check out books such as, 'Wheat Belly' by William Davis and 'The Paleo Diet' by Loren Cordain, 'Low Sugar No Sugar' by Jess Lomas, all contain menus, meal ideas and recipes. Go on-line and check out Nora's website www.primalbody-prinalmind.com.

*   *   *   *   *   *   *

Chapter 6

Fats - Saturated fat and cholesterol - not the

'big baddies' they are made out to be.

Saturated, Monounsaturated and Polyunsaturated Omega-3 and Omega-6 fats and Cholesterol are required by our bodies to stay healthy and function properly. We can live very well without carbohydrates but we won't last long without fat.

Our bodies were designed to handle natural sources of fat, even in high amounts which is why we have a gallbladder. Fat is needed for fat soluble vitamins A,D,E and K to be absorbed from our small intestine and utilised by our body. From birth nature tells us that fat is our body's fuel; breast milk is 54% saturated fat. Every cell in our body requires saturated fat. Our muscles, lungs, heart, bones, liver and immune system can't function without it. Our brain is 70 % fat and relies on cholesterol to function properly and to protect it from free-radicals. As we get older our cholesterol levels rise to cope with the body's increasing levels of damaging free-radicals. Cholesterol is so important to our body's function that all our cells have a way to make their own supply. If our brain doesn't get enough cholesterol the mechanism that fires our neurotransmitters is impaired and data processing and memory functions deteriorate. [viii] Low cholesterol levels are far more damaging to the body than high ones, too low and we invite dementia. Neurologist, David Perlmutter, MD, in his book 'Grain Brain', points out that by substantially limiting carbohydrates and increasing fats and protein we can reprogram our genes back to the factory setting we had at birth and become a mentally sharp, fat-burning machine once again.

The process of fat metabolism is called ketosis. This means our body is burning fat for energy rather than burning carbohydrates. When we burn fat for energy our body and all our vital organs, especially our heart and brain, thrive because they are getting the right kind of fuel with the vitamins, minerals and essential fatty acids they need.

Saturated fats and oils such as coconut oil, unsalted butter, ghee and organic lard, are good for cooking because they are very stable when moderately heated. Coconut oil has the added benefit of anti microbial properties that can protect us from disease. Extra virgin olive oil and sesame oil are the only other oils that can be moderately heated. Olive oil, like most nut oils, should only be consumed in small amounts as they have high levels of omega-6 and only small levels of omega-3. Olive oil for example has a ratio of approx. 11 omega-6 to 1 omega-3.[ix]

The best sources of omega-3 fatty acids are grass fed meats including organ-meat, and cold water fish and sea foods. Green leafy vegetables such as kale, avocados and walnuts are also a good source. Cod liver oil and krill oil go rancid very quickly so I don't recommend relying on them for your omega-3 fatty acids.

'Trans-fatty acids' (trans fats) are the fats to avoid. They are manufactured and completely unnatural, often labelled 'hydrogenated' or 'partially hydrogenated'. They are found in most commercial vegetable oils, all heated oils, margarines, fast food, pastries, salad dressing and all baked and packaged foods. Trans-fatty acids lower our good cholesterol levels, cause our tissues to lose beneficial omega-3 fatty acids, stop insulin doing its job properly and interfere with the body's immune system and enzyme functions. They are extremely damaging to our body and its DNA and once eaten it takes a very long time for our bodies to be rid of them.

It's a myth that eating fat will make you fat. Gaining weight has little to do with our dietary fat consumption, so long as it isn't the hydrogenated variety. Gaining weight has everything to do with our consumption of addictive carbohydrates. Likewise eating foods high in cholesterol has little to no impact on our body's cholesterol levels.

So remember:

'Natural Fat is our body's fuel'

'Cholesterol is its lubricant'

'We need BOTH to remain Healthy'

* * * * * * *

Chapter 7

Protein

We can't survive without protein. We need **'quality complete protein'**, that is protein with the essential amino acids that can't be made by our bodies. Again it is our grass-fed meat and poultry, fish, seafood and eggs that provide the most **'complete protein' in the ideal ratio of protein to fat that we require.**

Avoid meat from grain fed animals as the grain they consume increases the omega-6 and depletes the omega-3 fatty acids in their tissues. Their meat is not a good source of omega-3 for our diets.

Vegetables provide some protein but not the 'complete protein' our body needs and cannot make. Our digestive system is not meant for a vegetarian diet, we only have one stomach whereas vegetarian animals have more than one to efficiently access plant nutrients.   For us strict vegetarianism for life is a recipe for nutritional disaster.

It only takes a small amount of 'complete protein', in combination with adequate dietary fat, to have our bodies functioning properly. **Too much protein in the absence of fat is toxic** causing problems such as headaches, general malaise, extreme fatigue, cardiac dysfunction and for some people who followed the fat-free liquid protein diet of the late 1970's, death. "Eating protein without fat isn't a good idea and has never been a natural occurrence that our digestive systems have had to cope with".[x]

Consuming excessive amounts of protein means some of it will be converted to sugar and stored as fat. Limiting our protein intake is actually beneficial and doing so has been shown to decrease cell damage giving us anti-cancer and anti-aging abilities. Our body uses protein in an interesting way, when it is restricted it uses it for repair and maintenance and when there is a constant sufficient amount of good quality protein it becomes a signal for growth and reproduction, suggesting that as we get older we benefit from eating less protein.

So how much is just enough? Nora Gedgaudas in her book 'Primal Body, Primal Mind, tells us that a daily range of 45-50gms of protein for an adult of average weight and metabolic demands, to 80gms of protein for the leanest, most muscular, and most metabolically demanding athletes. This for most adults this equates to 0.8gms per kilogram of ideal body weight (eg: someone weighing 68kg x 0.8gms = 54gms of complete protein per day).[xi]

When trying to work out how much protein is in a steak, for example, guidelines can be found on internet sites that show food listed by protein content. Try: - Wikipedia.org, Healthaliciousness.com, Nutritionfoundation.org.nz. Also Nora's book 'Primal Body, Primal Mind', has a comprehensive list.

Here are a few examples:

Grams of protein per 100gms of -

Fillet Steak – 40gms

Mince Meat – 24gms

Lamb – 20 to 50gms

Pork – 25gms

Chicken – 30gms

Fish – 26gms

Hard Cheese – 25-27gms

Milk, Yogurt – 6gms

Nuts & Seeds – 33gms

The less fat found in or on the meat the higher the protein content will be per portion. 'Game meats' are a good example of this.

Growing children, teenagers and breast feeding women need a higher intake of 'good quality complete protein', but the older we get the less we need.

By eating just enough protein to meet our body's need for repair, basic maintenance and regeneration we can increase our life span and defer signs of aging.

* * * * * * *

Chapter 8

Weight Loss Why Dieting only works Short Term!

A visit to any supermarket shows that if your trolley is laden with food from the centre aisles your diet is going to be carbohydrate heavy. Breads, pastry, biscuits, muffins, cake, tinned fruit, jams, crisps, sweets, ice-cream, yoghurt, dips and sauces, potato chips, pasta, canned beans, spaghetti, fizzy drinks or juices, the list goes on. Also potatoes and kumera, like most vegetables grown below ground have a high starch content. All these carbohydrate, starch and sugar laden foods turn to glucose when eaten and if not used immediately are stored as fat.

If occasionally eaten as treats some of the above may well be harmless but eaten on a daily basis this level of carbohydrate consumption ensures weight gain and deterioration of our health. For some of us this shows up in our teens while for others, like me, not until my late 40's.

It never occurred to me that the quality of what I was eating was the cause of the excess weight around my middle. I thought it was more likely the quantity. I had always tried to keep to a fairly healthy diet, not too much meat - trimming the fat off, only whole grain bread, minimal desserts, fruit juices rather than alcohol and fruit rather than the chocolate bars I enjoyed in my teens. My exercise levels dropped as work and family took up more time. Fried food gave me indigestion so fish 'n' chips were never more than once or twice a month along with an occasional pizza and mango chicken as the only take-aways. I tried cutting down my food intake but by still eating the same foods nothing much happened, my weight kept creeping up. I was not what you would call highly over weight but the extra 6kgs I was carrying, mostly around my middle, made my clothes tight and me uncomfortable. I tired easily would get tearful and lethargic and my joints ached. I started to need glasses, my hair was brittle and thinning and I felt cold most of the time, I really felt like I was getting old. When I was mid way through my 50's I visited my doctor with my list of symptoms, I wasn't ready to be old. She tested my thyroid function and found it was below normal. I was relieved as this could be the answer. Fix my thyroid and I'd feel young again. I started taking some thyroid support herbs and iodine drops and yes I did feel a bit better but still I had aching joints, thinning hair and persistent excess weight.

About the same time I discovered a book called "Primal Body, Primal Mind", by Nora Gedgaudas which pointed out the course our eating trends had taken ever since we arrived on earth and how far removed our nutrition is today from our early ancestors. I did more research and read more books and came to the conclusion that what I was eating as my 'healthy diet' was far from it even though it was recommended by the country's Health Organisations and most food pyramids I found on the internet. I would need to change what I was eating and in my case go back to something close to what my parents ate when I was a youngster. This I thought I could do but it would mean one dinner for me and another for my partner that would double my work load, no way would I keep that up for long. But I was fortunate because my partner picked up Nora's book and got just as engrossed in it as I did. He was up for a change in diet too but not for weight loss. He felt annoyed at being fed so much 'garbage' over the years about what foods were supposedly good for him, when so many people were obviously suffering eating this recommended diet. He also wanted to reap the benefits of health and longevity going back to a natural fat burning diet would bring him.

So together we tried it. We followed Nora's recommendations and after only a month I was amazed at how much better I felt. I was effortlessly losing weight and I hadn't been restricting my food intake at all. My finger and knee joints weren't stiff in the mornings any more, my hair wasn't falling out when I combed it, I had way more energy and when I went back to the doctor to get my thyroid function tested again after three months it was back within normal range.

We gave up all grains, dairy and starchy vegetables for the first few months of our new way of eating but now after a year we have reintroduced some dairy and root vegetables but not potatoes. We enjoy our diet and have no desire to go back to eating breads, pastry, biscuits or cakes baked with flour (I use nut meal and make a fruit cake occasionally). Starting out with a hearty breakfast of eggs each morning we both find we have no cravings for carb laden foods. We both wish we had discovered the facts about our actual dietary requirements years ago.

If losing weight or regaining your health is what you want to achieve, start now!

Change the way and what you are eating starting with breakfast. (see suggested meal ideas)

Most diets only work for the short term. Initially with calorie restriction and exercise weight goes down but with our body's complex hormonal system restricting calories triggers a famine response. Our weight plateaus and then starts to rise again. The fat deposits reappear even when eating less of the same foods.

The resulting body fat produces excess hormones resulting in an imbalance within our body. Things start to go wrong and accessing enough of the right nutrients from our food even the healthy food doesn't happen. We get tired easily our blood glucose levels yo-yo and we gain more weight even though we try and eat less and exercise more.

Evolution has programmed our bodies to keep our weight stable or store, store, store in times of famine. Restricting food intake constitutes famine. Likewise excessive exercise signals to our body that we are in flight mode. Food will be scarce so hang on to what is there because something life threatening is happening which will need those reserves in the future in order to survive. Restrictive diets are really only a short term fix.

The key to sustained weight loss is this: If you restrict (or do away with) your 'carbohydrate intake' rather than your 'calorie intake' and replace those carbs with fat and protein, your body will regulate your weight for you and maintain your health.

Sounds simple, well 'yes' and 'no'. Carbohydrates and sugars are incredibly 'addictive', it requires strong will-power for the first few weeks but after that when you start to see and feel the difference it becomes easier, you won't want to go back to your old diet. Cutting out carbs completely is often more successful than cutting down.

Change the balance of what you are eating because it is the fat content of food that satisfies hunger and keeps you feeling full longer. Think – 'Higher fat/protein – Lower to no Carbs'. By fat I mean good fat, saturated, monounsaturated and polyunsaturated, in real terms that's meat with its fat on, eggs, avocados, nuts, sea food and fish, butter, coconut oil, coconut cream, raw full cream milk, cheese, plain unsweetened yoghurt. All these foods have the right ratio of fat to protein to completely satisfy hunger and stop addictive cravings. When eating sensibly fat doesn't make you fat. Eating carbohydrate does.

Be careful not to use corn, rice, tapioca or arrowroot flour in place of wheat flour because they are all very highly refined carbohydrates. Try using nut meal instead of flour. 'Wheat Belly' by William Davis, has a lovely recipe for an Apple and Walnut 'bread' using 2 cups of almond meal. I have also tried a similar recipe using half coconut meal and half almond. The other thing to look out for is added sugar and sugar substitutes. The fructose syrup versions will raise your blood glucose levels quicker and higher than ordinary table sugar.

* * * * * * *

Chapter 9

Eating our Way to a Healthy Body

Once you make the decision to change your diet you can find lots of helpful recipes and meal ideas on the internet or in some of these books:

"Low Carb Revolution" by Annie Bell – a wonderful cook book. At the time I bought my copy Amazon only had it for kindle. I sourced a copy from Scorpio Books, Christchurch.

"Low Sugar No Sugar" by Jess Lomas – great advice and recipes to start you off giving up sugar. Source it from Amazon or I found a copy in my local Library.

"The Paleo Diet" by Loren Cordain, Ph.D. – available from Amazon, it has a lot of insightful information as well as recipes. However Cordain has missed the point that Gedgaudas made about fat being the vital ingredient that curbs your hunger. Instead he believes it to be protein. Other research concurs with Gedgaudas so don't go for lean cuts, eat all fat in moderation. Cordain also has other cooks books available from Amazon.

"Wheat Belly" by William Davis, MD – 'lose the wheat, lose the weight'. A worthwhile book to read and it also includes helpful recipes. Available from Amazon.

"Primal Body, Primal Mind" by Nora Gedgaudas - Beyond the Paleo Diet for Total Health and Longer Life. A great reference book, available from Amazon. It also includes sample menus and if you go to her web site primalbody-primalmind.com, there are lots of recipes.

Here are some 'Simple Meal Ideas' and recommendations.

Breakfast:

Eggs: A nutrient rich food 62% fat 34% protein[xii]. Try slicing Eggplant and fry in a little coconut oil. When soft break 1 or 2 eggs over and continue cooking till eggs are done. Eggs scrambled or poached with onions and diced nitrate free bacon, fried tomato and mushrooms.

Homemade Muesli: Roughly chop a selection of raw nuts, add some lightly roasted coconut flakes and mix in a small amount of raisins or chopped dates. Take a small portion and spoon over some blueberries. Serve with plain yoghurt or coconut cream. (Roasting nuts degrades their nutrients and causes their fat/oils to go rancid)

Lunch:

Homemade vegetable soup: Made fresh or from left over vegetables from last night's dinner seasoned with herbs and spices, my favourite is a little curry powder and nutmeg then add some coconut milk.

Salad: A lovely mix of leafy greens with cucumber, avocado and tomato, a hand full of seeds and raw nuts, add some cold meat, tinned fish or homemade quiche.

Quiche: Again thin slices of egg plant make a good base, cover with slices of onion, smoked salmon, bacon or tuna, grated cheese, feta, cream cheese, sliced tomato, capsicums and mushrooms cover with beaten eggs and cook. Take a couple of slices cold with a salad.

Dinner:

Meat: From grass fed animals, cooked at a low heat for the shortest possible time to preserve all the nutrients. So this means eating steak rare and minimally cooking other meat where ever possible. Leftovers are great for lunch. "But meat is expensive", you say. Remember, you don't need at lot. Refer to the chapter on protein and work out how much you should be eating. Try some of the more interesting meats such as kidney, liver and heart. These meats are packed with the nutrients our bodies can access and they aren't expensive. They can also be very tasty when cooked with other meats making it all go further. Try a cheaper cut of steak chopped with kidneys, or thinly sliced liver cooked very quickly with bacon and mushrooms. Lamb's heart stuffed with herbs, onions and nuts then slow cooked, left to go cold, sliced thinly and put with a salad can make a great lunch.

Fish: Pan fried in a little olive oil or coconut oil, grilled or poached in coconut cream. Make a coating with egg and chopped nuts then lightly fry or grill. Poach and add to leek and kumera soup to make a quick seafood chowder.

Vegetables: Eat lots of leafy greens. Cabbage, kale, bok-choy and spinach are some good ones. Broccoli, cauliflower, brussel sprouts, green beans, leeks, celery, capsicums, mushrooms, pumpkin and many more. All root vegetables are quite starchy so only eat small quantities. Steam, stir-fry, lightly boil or roast. Never deep fry.

Salads: Eating vegetables raw is a good way of accessing their nutrients. Chop or grate them and add to leafy lettuce greens with a dressing of olive oil, balsamic or apple cider vinegar and a teaspoon of chunky mustard, tastes delicious.

Annie Bell in her book 'Low Carb Revolution' has several recipes for different delicious salad dressings.

Desserts:

Sometimes a necessary evil! Avoid anything with sugar and syrups. All fruit contains sugar in the form of fructose. Check out a glycaemic index (GI). It will tell you which fruits are very high and which are the more sensible ones to eat. Google search 'glycaemic index' and make yourself a copy. Use it as a guide when buying fruit and vegetables. For instance, most fresh fruit has a GI around 30, berries such as blackberries are 25, blueberries are believed to be about 3. Information on them is hard to find. Most nuts are about 15 whereas dried fruits are much higher, raisins about 64.

A sensible dessert could be: ½ a cup of blueberries with a couple of tablespoons of plain yoghurt and a dollop of coconut cream, sprinkled with grated almonds. You can also find coconut yoghurt and coconut ice-cream, but check out the added sugar, it would be pointless eating a no carb dinner then loading up on sugar for dessert.
'Bon Appetite'

Drinks:

Throw out your juicer and bring back all that fruit fibre your juicer discarded. By juicing fruit you are losing the nutrient rich fibre. Fibre also helps to slow down the digestive process avoiding that high fructose assault on your liver you get from drinking a glass of juice. Just a small glass of straight juice would give you a GI of 85.

So water it down and remember even liquid sugars gets converted to glucose and stored as fat.

Soy Milk – If you really want to poison yourself drink this stuff. Along with the other fashionable boxed milk substitutes found today, **don't go near them**. Read the ingredients and you will find you are drinking mostly canola oil, water, thickeners, and preservatives with a very small percentage of Soy, Rice, Oats, Almond, etc.

Soy, like wheat, contains the toxin phytic acid that blocks the uptake of essential minerals from food, promoting osteoporosis. It disrupts protein digestion and inhibits growth. **Soy has the highest phytic acid level of any of the grains or legumes and it isn't reduced by cooking.** It is also abundant in isoflavones, these are a class of phytoestrogens – plant compounds that mimic oestrogen. Isoflavones depress thyroid function. An underactive thyroid slows down your whole metabolism making it harder to lose weight. Drinking just two glasses of soy milk will do this for you. Another nasty hidden away in soy is a substance called haemaglutinin, a clot promoter that causes red blood cells to clump eventually clogging arteries[xiii]. Have I put you off yet?

Soy has become as invasive in our food as sugar and wheat. Soy flour is in almost all commercially made breads and confectionary. Read the ingredients and stop buying them.

A glass of water is probably the safest and healthiest drink you will find, drink cold or heat to make lots of lovely **herbals teas,** my favourites are liquorice, peppermint and refreshing green tea. Green tea is reported to be full of antioxidants that help to protect our cells from aging.

Coffee: Ummmm! It is a stimulant so keep it to one or two cups a day max. Pure Arabica coffee is reported to be naturally lower in caffeine so would be a good choice.

Decaffeinated coffee: The further from the original source you get the more toxins you incur. Decaffeination can be done using water but this also includes formic acid. Most decaffeination is done with solvents such as ethylacetate, methylene chloride, dichloromethane or supercritical $CO2$. Residues remain and although there are strict limits by law for those amounts, by drinking decaffeinated coffee you are adding toxins into your body for your liver to deal with. Every drink promotes glycation helping to age you, so decaffeinated coffee is not a good choice.

Black Tea: Also contains caffeine at about half the amount of coffee. Both coffee and tea should not be drunk with a meal as they hinder the absorption of nutrients. Also drinking liquid at or straight after a meal dilutes stomach acid making it harder to digest food.

Milk: We were designed to drink human milk up to the ages of 2 to 5 years at which time we stop producing the enzyme lactase needed to digest lactose – milk sugar. We were never designed to drink cow's milk, some of us tolerate it but 75% of the world's population is dairy intolerant. Drinking or eating dairy increases the body's level of insulin-like growth factor-1 (IGF1) which is a known cancer promoter.[xiv] There is no scientific evidence that dairy prevents osteoporosis - it may in fact promote bone loss. The calcium in milk is not readily accessible to our bodies so drinking milk to increase bone strength is a fallacy. In fact consuming less dairy and insuring adequate Vit.D from sunlight, is more important to bone health.[xv] 85% of milk is made up of casein - milk protein, which is a known promoter of cancer growth in all stages.[xvi]

The designer milks and fat reduced products sold today are not healthy and have been linked to changes in blood-fat chemistry which cause heart disease. Our bodies can deal with the fat molecules of whole milk in a normal digestive manner but once the milk has been altered and/or homogenised the fat molecules become smaller enabling them to pass into areas of the body where they are not welcome, triggering auto-immune diseases, allergies, asthma, irritable bowel and nutrient deficiencies.

If I haven't put you off yet then Raw- whole organic milk bought in a glass bottle or made into cheese and yogurt, should be your only choice. It won't contain the pesticide residues, PCB's, added hormones and antibiotics the widespread commercial brands do. You can get all your calcium from dark green leafy vegetables, sea vegetables and sea foods, sardines, salmon, grass fed meats and vit.D from sunshine. By not taking calcium supplements and seriously cutting down or eliminating dairy you won't be putting your body at risk of calcium depletion leading to osteoporosis. You will feel better, have clearer sinuses, fewer headaches, not experience the effects of irritable bowel and have more energy and less weight gain.

Alcohol: Has no nutritional value and very quickly metabolises into fat. It is addictive, stimulates insulin production in the same way carbohydrates and sugar do. It is reported that an occasional glass of wine (4-7% fructose) could assist in clearing fats from our arteries but chronic (consistent) alcohol consumption leads to liver damage.[xvii]

Moderation is the key but if you suffer from any autoimmune disease alcohol will only make it worse as it behaves in the same way the lectins in all grains and legumes do which is to increase intestinal permeability giving you a leaky-gut.[xviii]   Alcohol sugars have a delayed glycaemic effect which is often why after an evening out drinking you feel shaky the next day.

Nuts and Seeds: Excellent to snack on but don't overdo them. Eat no more than a handful a day. Nuts provide us with omega-3 and 6, walnuts having higher levels of omega-3. Brazil's are a good source of selenium. Most nuts will contribute significant amounts of iron, zinc and magnesium if just a few are eaten daily.

Sugar: It should be classified as a **'Poison'** and come with a warning.

The consumption of any sugar, white, brown, raw, castor, fructose or golden syrup, corn syrup, high fructose corn syrup, maple syrup, malt, molasses, honey, glucose, dextrose, maltodextrin, agave, etc, etc, and all the sugar substitutes, cause a host of illnesses. High fructose corn syrup has proved to be the most addictive and damaging of all the sweeteners.

Some of the illnesses linked to sugar are; tooth decay, high blood pressure, diabetes, blindness, gout, inflammation, nerve damage, fatty liver, cirrhosis of the liver, liver failure, acute pancreatitis, kidney disease, polycystic ovary syndrome, stroke, obesity, ADHD, dementia, Alzheimer's, depression and anxiety.[xix]

Our primal ancestors never got the opportunity to consume large amounts of either sugar or carbohydrates and this shows itself in the fact that our bodies have several hormones designed to raise our glucose levels but only one that can actually lower it, and today it is vastly over worked.

Personally I believe sugary treats to be the most addictive substances on the planet. I am still battling to give them up completely. Because I am older and have started to feel the effects of what I have been consuming over the years I am finding it easier to listen to my wake-up call.

Food manufactures started adding sugar to products because they found people bought more. In 1945 a quarter of the sugar we ate was already in our food when we bought it, now days it's as high as three quarters. High fructose corn syrup, often labelled corn syrup or just syrup, accounts for a great deal of this. It is found in soft drinks, drink syrups, juices, biscuits, soups, yogurt, food dressings, health bars, and most processed foods. Fruit juice, which was thought to be a healthy alternative to fizzy soft drinks, is definitely not – "Before you have even finished your glass of apple juice, the fructose in the first mouthful will be circulating in your bloodstream as... (triglycerides)" [xx] and soon after deposited as fat in your cells.

Most sugars are a combination of glucose and fructose, each of these are dealt with differently by our bodies. Glucose triggers our pancreas to produce insulin which then takes the glucose from the blood stream and stores it as fat in the tissues of our muscles, liver and around our waist. Fructose goes straight to our liver, spiking our cortisol levels and is turned into glycogen and stored as fat. Some of this fat is used as fuel but most remains as fat. Our diets today are overloading our bodies with sugar rich foods spiking our insulin and cortisol levels way beyond healthy limits and over loading our liver and other organs with fat. **High insulin levels and high**

amounts of sugar staying in the blood stream leads to type 2 diabetes.

Fructose, along with being highly addictive also has the ability to disrupt our body's natural appetite regulator - leptin, leading us to over consumption and obesity.

The only way to completely avoid sugar is to go back to basics, avoid processed foods and prepare our food from scratch so we know exactly what is in it.

The lower we can maintain our blood sugar levels the less insulin and cortisol we produce, the slower glycation occurs, the healthier we remain and the longer we live.

Jess Lomas, in her book 'Low Sugar No Sugar', puts is beautifully by saying - "Sugar is an addiction that starts young and stays with us throughout life...a Low Sugar No Sugar lifestyle takes time, patience and perseverance. The world is against you at every turn, tempting you to fall back on old ways...".[xxi]

I couldn't agree with her more. Our bodies have no defence and the only way out is our own resolve. Try making nuts a snack food alternative, along with the occasional fig or date, raw celery and carrot sticks or slices of cucumber. Once you get used these they are really great.

*   *   *   *   *   *   *

Chapter 10

"Are Healthy Whole Grains Killing Us?"

The answer is indisputably 'YES'.

So much evidence of grain especially wheat's link to modern illnesses can be seen all around us once we open our eyes. Opting for a low fat diet that minimized cholesterol and glorified grains started this decline in our health. Just because wheat related illnesses have become more common doesn't make them a normal part of aging. This I can personally vouch for as my overall health improved remarkably after I stopped eating grains. So to sum it all up:

Grains and Grain-like Seeds to avoid:

Wheat, Barley, Corn, Oats, Rice, Wild Rice, Rye, Sorghum, Millet, Amaranth, Buckwheat, Quinoa and all products containing any amount of these.

Today's Wheat: A super carbohydrate with high gluten levels leading not only to type II Diabetes, Coeliac disease and Leaky Gut Syndrome but also inflammation throughout the body causing Neurological illnesses such as Headaches, Depression, Epilepsy, Schizophrenia, Autism, ADHD, Dementia and Alzheimer's.[xxii]

Remember today's wheat may be the worst offender but **all grains** have the same ability to make us sick because they contain:

Phytates: Bind with minerals making them unavailable to us, depriving and depleting our bodies of calcium – leading to osteoporosis, iron, magnesium and zinc.

Goitrogens: Thyroid inhibiting substances causing underactive thyroid function.

Exphorins: Morphine like compounds that cause cravings for more carbohydrates - more bread, more cake, more biscuits, etc. etc. etc.

Gluten: Doesn't just affect our digestive tract as in Celiac Disease and give us food allergies but it affects our brain, heart, kidneys, nervous system and immune system. Gluten sensitivity is a silent killer more common than we give it credit for and a number one cause of inflammation through-out our bodies.[xxiii] Responsible for brain fog – confusion, depression and anxiety, ADHD, dementia and Alzheimer's, gluten's role in the decline of our health is screaming at us. We need to start now and **stop eating all grains.**

Remember **be aware of any food labelled 'Gluten Free'**. Read that label carefully to make sure it doesn't contain any grain and hasn't substituted soy, rice, corn, tapioca etc. for wheat flour, all of which are highly refined carbohydrates which overload us with glucose.

Listen to Nora Gedgaudas when she tells us that any grain consumption isn't worth the dietary risk because - **"there is no one alive for whom grains of any type are essential for health, and gluten, in particular, is a health food for no one."** [xxiv]

To live a long and active life we need to watch what we eat and not be seduced by advertising. Remember "Healthy Whole Grains", not true! Buy fresh! If you have to check the label for additives then it's not going to be good for you. Take control of your diet and you control your future. Don't leave it up to others. Question everything, from the food you buy to the advice of your health practitioner. You only have one life and one body so make the most of it for as long as you can.

* * * * * * *

Chapter 11

Recipes – here are a few of my favourites

Nut Flours: Substituting nut flours for wheat flour can work well but will never be quite as light and fluffy.

Nut flours (the same as nuts) should only be eaten in moderation because although they contain beneficial omega-3 fatty acids they are high in omega-6 of which we only need small amounts.

I will start by giving you my special occasion boiled fruit cake recipe. It is quick and easy to make and gives me something to offer guests that we can eat as well, but it pays to check for any nut allergies before handing it around.

Quick and Easy Boiled Fruit Cake

Two handfuls of Raisins, Two handfuls of chopped Dates, One large chopped Banana, One small diced Pear, Juice of one Mandarin, Two tablespoons of extra virgin olive oil.

Put all of the above in a saucepan and just cover with water and bring to the boil, simmer for a couple of minutes, turn off and let cool.

Beat three eggs and stir into cool mix and add one to two cups of almond flour/meal and a half cup of coconut flour, I have also used walnut flour. ½ tsp baking soda.

The mix should be moist, not too stiff or too runny but pourable. Pour into cake tin lined with baking paper. Bake for approx 50mins in medium temp. oven. When cold cut into cubes eat immediately or store in cool place.

Blueberry Banana Breakfast Smoothy - for two

Combine half a cup of fresh or frozen Blueberries, one Banana, one can (270mls) Coconut cream, in blender and blend on high until smooth and creamy, add a little water or ice cubes if too thick.

Quick Cooked Breakfast – for one

Slice two to three rounds of Eggplant and place in hot fry pan with a little coconut oil, sear both sides then turn heat down, add more coconut oil, put lid on and cook till soft. Add two eggs and continue cooking till eggs are done but yolks still soft. Serve or eat straight out of pan.

Pumpkin and Spinach Soup – Jess Lomas, *"Low Sugar No Sugar"*

300g Pumpkin diced and skin removed, 2tbsp Coconut oil, 4 cups Chicken or vege stock, 200g Baby Spinach, 1 cup Coconut cream, salt and pepper to taste.

Combine pumpkin and coconut oil along with a tsp of chilli flakes (ginger, cumin, nutmeg, or turmeric could be substituted for the chilli) and roast in oven for 23-30mins. In saucepan combine stock, roasted pumpkin and baby spinach. Bring to a simmer for 5 mins, cool and blend, stir through coconut cream and season.

Kumera Salmon Hash Cakes – great for lunches

210g can of Atlantic Salmon, 2 cups diced Kumera, 3 Eggs, 1/2 cup grated Cheese, handful of chopped Parsley.

Boil Kumera till slightly soft. Drain, cool, then add other ingredients, mix thoroughly, spoon evenly into muffin tin, sprinkle each with a little more grated cheese. Cook till set and golden around 15mins at 180 C.

Casserole Baked Lamb Neck Chops – for two

Put 4 Lamb neck Chops in a casserole dish with 2 tbsp Coconut Oil and ¼ cup water. Sprinkle over with rubbed rosemary. Slice up two medium onions and two parsnips and place around the meat. Cover and bake on low to medium for 1/2 hr, checking it's not drying out. Serve with cauliflower mash, steamed broccoli and bok choy.

Liver and Bacon – Yes it is very nice – serves 4.

450gm approx of thinly sliced Lambs Liver, 2 tbsp coconut oil, 1 large onion sliced, 2 cloves of garlic minced, 6 (or more if you prefer) slices of nitrate free bacon chopped.

Heat 1tbsp coconut oil in fry pan and add onion, garlic and bacon, cook till onion browns, put aside and heat the other tbsp of coconut oil in fry pan and lightly sear the thin slices of liver, don't overcook. Combine all back in pan and heat through, serve. Goes well with cauliflower mash and steamed vegetables.

Cauliflower Mash - Basically just boiled or steamed then mashed cauliflower, a great substitute for mash potato. The various types of cauliflower available make for a colourful dish, white, green or purple.

Kale Chips – I found these in a few recipe books, here is my version.

3-4 storks of washed and dried kale, storks removed and kale torn into small pieces, place in a bowl with ¼ cup extra virgin olive oil and a very small amount of salt and pepper you can always add more later. Rub oil into kale until well covered. Lay out on a baking tray lined with baking paper and cook on medium heat for approx 30mins or until edges are just turning a light brown and kale has dried out, very easy to overdo so keep an eye on them. Delicious!

Avocado and Tomato Salsa – great as a dip with cucumber rounds or on own with a salad or as an accompaniment to a fish dish.

1 Avocado diced, 1 Large Tomato diced, 1 Tbsp Extra Virgin Olive Oil, 1 Tbsp Apple Cider Vinegar, 1 tsp course mustard.

Combine avocado and tomato in a bowl, separately combine oil, vinegar and mustard and mix well. Then pour small quantity over avocado and tomato and mix in. Serve.

Pizza Base – this I also found in a few recipe books and think it's great, hope you love it too.

1 small head of cauliflower grated and steamed for a very short time, well drained, a hand full of grated cheese, 1 egg, and a little salt and pepper.

Mix all together in bowl then press thin and even into a pizza size tray. Bake for about 30mins, until firm and edges are slightly golden brown. Now add your topping.

My favourite is some freshly cooked salmon, small dollops of cream cheese combined with a sprinkling of feta cheese, some chopped olives, some pre cooked chopped broccoli and finely chopped red onion, a sprinkling of course mustard. Put under grill for approx. 5mins then add a few baby spinach leaves before serving.

Eggs – Boiled halved and yolks mixed with a little butter, yoghurt, curry powder, salt and pepper, spooned back into the halves and you have yummy curried eggs.

Wraps – Annie Bell – *"Low Carb Revolution"*

4 eggs, 1 Tbsp Extra Virgin Olive Oil, 1 Tbsp Water, Salt and Pepper to taste.

Mix thoroughly, spread 2 -3 spoons thinly in fry pan, cook as for pancakes. Leave to cool, then fill with cooked chicken and salad, smoked salmon and cream cheese, avocado and tomato, etc .

Wraps can be made in advance and stored in cool place without fillings to use the next day.

Peach Mousse

2 Sheets of Gelatine, 1 410g tin of Peaches in juice not syrup – drained , 1 270g tin of Coconut Cream, Whites of two Eggs beaten till nearly stiff.

In a bowl blend the drained peaches and stir in the coconut cream. Soak the gelatine in cold water, drain and pour 2Tbsp hot water over sheets to melt them. Whisk them into the peach mix. Lastly fold the beaten eggs whites into mixture. Carefully spoon mix into small serving bowls and refrigerate for at least 4 hours.

Nutty Fudge Bites - a version of a recipe by Jess Lomas - *"Low Sugar No Sugar"*

1 cup of Almond Butter, ½ cup Coconut Oil, ½ cup Cocoa powder, ½ cup chopped Cashew nuts.

Melt coconut oil and mix thoroughly into nut butter and cocoa powder. Roughly chops cashew nuts and fold into mix. Pour into lined tray, sprinkle with shredded coconut and refrigerate, cut into small squares and store in fridge.

Renata's scrummy muesli nibbles

Take a selection of your favourite nuts, ½ cup of each. Roughly chop and mix together in bowl with:

1 Tbsp honey,   1Tbsp coconut oil – melted

1 tsp cinnamon

Spread evenly on a baking paper covered oven tray.

Bake in oven 100-150 C for approx 10-12mins, turning frequently until light brown. Leave to cool and store in air tight container in the fridge.

For a non honey version, when cold, add a handful of raisins or chopped dates, figs or dried blueberries.

(Remember by heating the nuts you are losing some of their nutrients and degrading their oils, so this should not be an everyday food but rather a treat!)

Another web site worth looking at for more delicious recipes that follow a low-carb, gluten-free, and like-minded way of eating is www.primalbody-primalmind.com.

And check out Danielle Walker's cook books 'Against all Grains'- well worth buying.

*   *   *   *   *   *   *

References

i   Petit, J.R., Jouzel, J., Raynaud, D., et al. "Climate and Atmospheric History of the Past 420,000 Years from the Vostok Ice Core, Antarctica," *Nature* 399, no. 6735 (1999): 429-36.

ii Gedgaudas, N.T. 2009-11. *Primal Body, Primal Mind.* Healing Arts Press; 1:7. Canada.

iii Leonard, W.R., et al. 2003. "Metabolic Correlates of Hominid Brain Evolution*" Comparative Biochemistry and Physiology Part A: Molecular & Integrative Physiology* 136: 5-15.

iv Davis, W. MD. 2011. *Wheat Belly.* Roydale Books, Macmillian, USA.

v   Rosedale, R. January 13, 2008. "Insulin, Leptin, Diabetes, and Aging: Not So Strange Bedfellows." *Diabetes Health.* www.diabeteshealth.com/read/2008/01/13/5617.html.

vi Davis, W. MD. 2011. *Wheat Belly.* Roydale Books, Macmillian, USA.

vii Perlumutter, D. 2013. *Grain Brain.* Little, Brown and Company. USA.

viii Gedgaudas, N.T. 2009-11. *Primal Body, Primal Mind.* Healing Arts Press; 21:200. Canada.

ix Gedgaudas, N.T. 2009-11. *Primal Body, Primal Mind.* Healing Arts Press; 21:196,197. Canada.

x   Cordain L, Ph.D. 2011. *The Paleo Diet Cookbook.* Wiley. 1:16. USA.

xi Fallon, S. and Enig, M. Lifstyle Autum 2002. 97-101. NZ. (Sally Fallon is a Nutritional Scientist and President of the 'Weston A Price Foundation'), 1999. www.westonaprice.org

Disclaimer

Any use of the information I have provided in my book is your personal choice. It is not intended to serve as a total replacement for professional medical advice. It is intended as an informational guide only and should not be used to treat a serious ailment without first consulting with a qualified health care professional.

Acknowledgments

Grateful thanks to my partner, who tirelessly read and re read my notes and helped with research. It has been an enjoyable journey made more so by his participation. Many thanks to my friend Paula for her help with proof reading. Also a big thank you to all my family and friends who have listened to these ideas, I wish you many long healthy years.

[xii] Hyman M, MD. Dairy: 6 reasons you should avoid it at all costs. Huffingtonpost.com; Healthy living: Oct 14, 2014.

[xiii] Feskanich D, Willett WC, Stampfer MJ, Colditz GA. Milk, dietary calcium and bone fracture in women: a 12 year prospective study. AMJ Public Health.1977 Jun;87(6):992-7.

[xiv] Huncharek M, Muscat J, Kupelnick B. Colerectal cancer risk and dietary intake of calcium, vit D and dairy products: a meta-analysis of 26,335 cases from 60 observational studies. Nutr Cancer. 2009;61(1):47-69.

[xv] Gillespie D. 2010. *The Sweet Poison Quit Plan.* Viking Penguin Group. Australia.

[xvi] Cordain L, Ph.D. 2011. *The Paleo Diet*, revised edition. Wiley and Sons Inc. USA.

[xvii] Perlmutter D, MD. 2013. *Grain Brain*. Little, Brown and Company. 1:29. USA.

[xviii] Gillespie D. 2010. *The Sweet Poison Quit Plan.* Introduction; 17. Viking Penguin Group. Australia.

[xix] Lomas J. 2014. *Low Sugar No Sugar*. Wilkinson Publishing Pty Ltd. Australia.

[xx] Perlmutter D, MD. 2013. *Grain Brain*. Little, Brown and Company. 1:32. USA.

[xxi] Gedgaudas, N.T. 2009-11. *Primal Body, Primal Mind.* Healing Arts Press; 3:29. Canada.

[xxii] Gedgaudas, N.T. 2009-11. *Primal Body, Primal Mind.* Healing Arts Press; 3:48. Canada.

www.ingramcontent.com/pod-product-compliance
Lightning Source LLC
Chambersburg PA
CBHW060649290526
45793CB00001B/456